BETTY

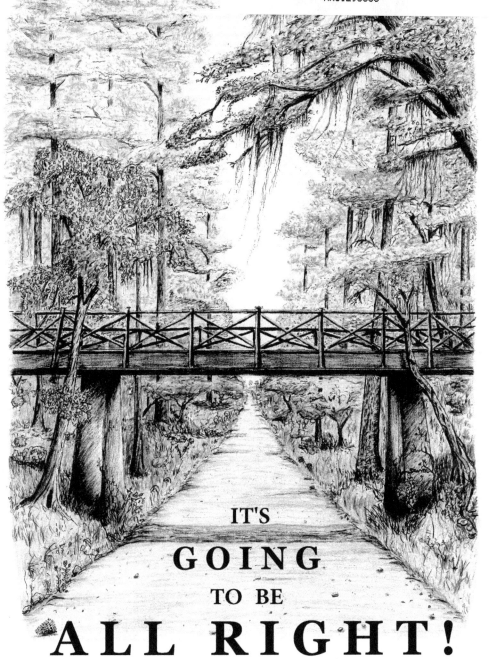

IT'S GOING TO BE ALL RIGHT!

A Collection of Positive Reflections

outskirts press

Outskirts Press, Inc.
http://www.outskirtspress.com

Paperback ISBN: 978-1-9772-0252-9
Hardback ISBN: 978-1-9772-0226-0

Cover Illustration by Richard Sawyer
Author Photo by Andy Shivers

Outskirts Press and the "OP" logo are trademarks belonging to Outskirts Press, Inc.

PRINTED IN THE UNITED STATES OF AMERICA

"Betty and I have been close friends for many years. I am always impressed by her positive attitude. I admire her ability to influence others with her enthusiasm. This book will help people."

The Late Jean Morgan Hathaway,
Former Member, Board of Directors, Archbold Medical Center

"The true epitome of a Southern lady! This inspiring collection of her thoughts will bring you comfort."

Jimmy Singletary,
Business Owner, Singletary Flowers & Gifts

"My dear friend, Betty Sawyer, has impacted the Thomasville community in many ways. She is a kind and gentle person who loves to share her extensive knowledge and experience with others. She is highly motivated and deeply committed to helping others."

Dr. Steve DePaola,
Associate Professor of Psychology, Thomas University

"Thank you, Betty Sawyer, for being an awesome friend and mentor as I walked this dark road learning the art of Alzheimer's disease. You have been there for our family every step of the way. You have taught me so much about dealing with the emotions associated with this disease."

Kathy Megahee,
Executive Director, Thomas County Family Connection

"Betty Sawyer...an extraordinary lady full of love for her family, friends, and community. Her words of inspiration and delightful wit are sure to bless and reassure you that "It's going to be all right."

DEDICATION

This book is dedicated to the most loving family any mother, grandmother, or great-grandmother could have. I have felt cherished, respected, protected, admired, and loved every day. I am thankful for each of you.

Table of Contents

Foreword

Everybody needs a hero. Webster's defines 'hero' as "a person who is admired or idealized for courage, achievements, or noble qualities." A synonym for 'hero' is 'Betty Sawyer' – and I don't need a thesaurus to tell me that. The author of this book is my hero – but she is also a hero to many others. Reading this book will give you, the reader, an opportunity to bask in the positivity that Betty radiates. She truly is the most positive person I've ever known.

Betty's late husband, Walt, who had dementia, was one of the first residents of Plantation Manor Assisted Living Community where I served as Executive Director. Betty had retired several years earlier from an impressive career as a social worker with the State of Georgia, to care for Walt at home. She volunteered her time at our community and quickly became an invaluable member of our family.

After Walt passed away, we asked Betty to come onboard as our Director of Social Services. Thankfully, she agreed. She jumped headfirst into her new role and never looked back. Her devotion and dedication to our residents, their families, and our staff members were boundless. In addition to her regular duties, Betty set about organizing the Alzheimer's/Dementia

Family Caregiver Support Group. Under her leadership, the group continued to grow and thrive. In 2007, Betty received the prestigious Horizons Award from the Alzheimer's Association of Georgia for her work with the group, "the largest & most consistently well-attended caregiver support group in the state." The group continues today (with Betty's guidance) and has helped hundreds of people cope with the grief and stressors which are a regular part of the journey that is Alzheimer's.

Betty also continues to serve as Ambassador of Legacy Village at Plantation Manor (although she retired for the second time in 2015, after 14 years of service to that wonderful community). I served with her for 12 of those years -- and I make no secret of the fact that I could not have succeeded in my role without Betty. Even though I was (technically) her supervisor, it was she who advised me, comforted me and inspired me. She was my mentor, my friend, and my hero. If I had a dollar for every time Betty told me, "It's going to be all right," I would be a wealthy woman today.

Betty has worked tirelessly in the fight against Alzheimer's/ dementia. In 2006, she initiated the Walter Sawyer Memorial Day Program which made a positive difference in the lives of the many attendees as well as their loved ones. She served for many years on the planning committee of the Jim Neill Walk for Alzheimer's Awareness and the Jim Neill Foundation. Betty volunteered extensively with the Alzheimer's Association of Southwest Georgia and has been very involved with the Red Hills Gerontology Association. I could go on and on -- but I think you get the idea. Betty's selfless devotion to others is boundless. Her grace, charm, and humor make her a sought-after speaker as well as an excellent writer.

I would be remiss if I failed to mention Betty's faith in God. She has never made any bones about the fact that He is the source of her strength, her unfailing positivity, and her boundless love for others. Betty Sawyer is 87 years old. She is the most energetic, engaged, supportive person I know -- and, did you get that, she is 87!!!!

You, dear reader, are blessed to have this book in your hands. When you have finished reading it, you will know that it really is going to be all right. You will also know why Betty Sawyer is my hero – and I'll bet she will be your hero, too.

Gail Lancaster
Executive Director
Oaks at Hampton (Assisted Living Community)

Acknowledgments

The incredible artwork on the cover is entitled *The South of Thomasville*. It was drawn by my son, Richard Sawyer, for which I am extremely grateful. Thanks so much to my editor, Sue Keith, and to my precious granddaughter, Ansley Ragan Evans, for typing the manuscript. Thanks also to my dear friend, Gail Lancaster, for the Foreword, and my daughter, Beth Sawyer Ragan, for the lovely Afterword.

Introduction

Some people might say the age of 87 is too old to write your first book. I disagree! My life has been filled with so much joy and laughter, as well as some pain and some tears, but mostly happiness. Therefore, I am anxious to share with you my philosophy, my feelings, and my faith.

All my life I have loved words – using words, reading words, and writing words. I am fascinated by their ability to move, change, and inspire people. By the way, people are a favorite of mine too! I am often described as a "people person," which I consider a great compliment.

My purpose in writing this book, therefore, is to use words to make a difference in the lives of people. I have been in the helping profession of social work for over 45 years, so it is natural for me to want to be a positive influence whenever and however I can. I always say to each member of my family, or a friend who is going through a crisis, difficulty or problem, "It's going to be all right." Because that is what I have always believed, it is the reason my book title became "It's Going To Be All Right."

CHAPTER ONE

Early History

My life began precariously. I was born August 13, 1931, in Atlanta, Georgia. Weighing only three pounds, my chances of survival were slim. My parents, Doris Amanda Whitaker Spell and Cecil Emory Spell, were more concerned at the time with my mother's health. She was severely ill when I was born. In 1931, care for premature infants was not widely available, so for me, it was a dresser drawer for a bed and lots of prayers. Amazingly, I thrived, and although I was small, I became a very healthy child. I enjoyed boundless love from all my family members, especially from my daddy, who was my favorite. I grew up happy and secure.

When I was seven, we moved from Atlanta to Valdosta, Georgia. I graduated from high school and college in Valdosta, never leaving home until the day I married. Through my college years, and after graduation, I enjoyed my childhood friends, the "Big 9," as we called ourselves. It was a close and remarkable group – we were friends all through grade school, adolescence and into our adult lives. All of us were college graduates and all of us who married never divorced. I was a bridesmaid in seven weddings. I enjoyed an active social life with my friends and was engaged several times before actually getting married to my husband at the age of twenty-five!

From an early age around five or six until my early twenties, I had a problem that was unmistakable. I was very, very underweight. "Skinny" would be the best description. What made it easier to tolerate was people would say, "Betty Jean has the prettiest face; it is a shame she is so thin!" I chose to focus on the pretty face part. My weight finally stabilized after I married and became pregnant. I no longer have the problem of being too skinny!

CHAPTER TWO

The Good Life

I met my husband, Walter Sawyer, on a blind date. He was from Cairo, Georgia, and at the time, a loan manager in Valdosta. I was working for a radiologist in Valdosta at the time. After we married, we moved to Savannah, Georgia, where my husband had accepted a new position. I began working with a local radiologist, after receiving the highest praise and recommendation from my former employer. When I became pregnant, I was so ill that I spent every day prostrate on his X-ray table! I was not the grand employee my former boss had recommended!

From Savannah, my husband and I moved several more times until landing permanently in Thomasville, Georgia. By this time we had two children, Beth, our oldest, and Richard, our son. They began their school years in our new town. From the beginning I loved Thomasville; it is a lovely place filled with friendly and charming people. In April 1965, I found an article in the *Thomasville Times-Enterprise* newspaper that was of great interest to me. The Mental Health Clinic was opening at Archbold Medical Center. I met with Thomas County Health Commissioner, the late Dr. Joseph I. Palmer, who was directing the project. I was hired immediately as the social worker for the clinic, which included patients from Thomas, Grady and Brooks counties. I learned so much in that position by handling intakes, compiling social histories, and assisting with supportive counseling. I enjoyed learning under the supervision of the late Dr. Jack May, Clinical Psychologist. However, I was presented with a new opportunity.

The late Jean Morgan Hathaway, a former Board of Trustees' member of Archbold Medical Center, offered me the position of Social Worker at the newly formed Thomas-Grady Service Center, where she served as the director at the time. The service center provides adults with developmental disabilities opportunities to discover their gifts and realize their hopes and dreams through advocacy. By 1970, I found myself visiting the homes of prospective clients in every corner of Thomasville and Grady counties. Working with families with adults and children with special needs and learning disabilities was a privilege for me. I also taught the home-bound students who were unable to come to the facility. I learned a lot from each case I handled.

I retired in 1995, thirty years from the day I began. I had gained valuable knowledge and experience. However, even as a retiree, I was destined to continue learning on a more personal level.

CHAPTER THREE

Life's Challenges

My retirement began smoothly. I adored my two grandchildren, Ansley Ragan Evans and Amanda Ragan Ritter, as my life revolved around them. By the time I retired, my daughter Beth and her husband, Allen Ragan, had moved to Americus, Georgia, taking my two loves with them. However, the move did not prevent me from spending a great deal of time with them. Between visits back and forth to Americus, I shopped and "did lunch" with friends and thoroughly enjoyed my retirement. Several years after I retired, I began to notice my husband, Walt, having mood swings and at times, becoming increasingly aggressive.

Walt was happy one minute and depressed the next; his behavior evolved into extreme paranoia. His unwarranted jealousy affected every aspect of our lives. After extensive doctors' visits and tests, his diagnosis was Dementia with Lewy Body disease (DLB). According to the Alzheimer's Association's definition, this type of progressive dementia leads to a decline in thinking, reasoning, and independent function, because of abnormal microscopic deposits that damage brain cells over time. DLB closely resembles the symptoms of Alzheimer's disease and Parkinson's disease. Hallucinations are common with DLB, as are sleep problems and behavioral problems.

During extremely stressful times, joyous events happen as well. Richard and Kristan, my son and daughter-in-law, brought their baby son, Aaron Emory Sawyer, into our lives on May 10, 2000. Walt was happiest when holding or playing with Aaron.

By sheer determination, I was able to care for my husband at home for over five years. Of course, his condition deteriorated steadily, and in 2001, I was forced to move him to an assisted living facility. God gave me the strength to keep him at home for that period *and* to take the necessary step when the time came. I, along with my daughter, Beth, searched for the best living situation for him. I felt as though God was leading me in this choice.

In January, 2002, Walt moved into Plantation Manor's assisted living community. This move began a new chapter in both of our lives. Walt adjusted well at Plantation Manor and I decided to volunteer at the facility to be near him. Inevitably, his illness progressed and he passed away on July 5, 2002.

Because it has always been my nature to find something positive in an unfortunate situation, I wanted to do something to honor Walt. Searching for that "something" became the way I was able to grieve the loss of my kind and gentle husband. As I prayed for guidance, I continued to volunteer at Plantation

Manor. By this time, my volunteer work had evolved into the position of Director of Social Work for the facility.

As I was praying one night, I received an answer to my question of how to honor my beloved husband. I decided to start a support group for families in the Thomasville area who were dealing with a loved one with dementia, especially the most prevalent type of dementia, that of Alzheimer's disease. With the full support of our Executive Director at the time, Gail Lancaster, the first meeting of the Alzheimer's/ Dementia Support Group was at Plantation Manor in January of 2003.

God richly blessed this group from the very beginning. We began meeting in the upstairs dining room and served lunch to the group members. We quickly outgrew that location, as well as the next one in the building, and eventually, there were so many attendees we could no longer provide lunch. Our third and final meeting place became the center of Plantation Manor, the large living room on the first floor. Our membership grew to eighty-eight members with an average attendance of forty-five to fifty participants each month.

In 2007, I received the Horizon Award for outstanding volunteers from the Georgia Chapter of the Alzheimer's Association for my work with the group. The award is very special to me. For several years, our group was the largest and most well attended in the state of Georgia. I learned so much as I experienced the challenge of caring for a loved one with dementia. I will never know how one goes through this experience without God's help. His love surrounded me every minute and He gave me the strength to meet every day with confidence.

During my work at Plantation Manor, I was asked to write articles for the *Thomasville Times-Enterprise* newspaper's quarterly magazines, "Health Matters" and "Senior Living." I continued writing for the publication after my retirement. The next few chapters in this book include some of my most requested topics and newspaper articles, edited with updated information.

CHAPTER FOUR

An Extra Special Blessing

We all know how awesome becoming a grandparent can be. Well, if you think that is special, wait until you become a great-grandparent! This experience is awe-inspiring. If your grandchild is treasured in your life, how amazing that child's child will be!

After my great-grandson was born, just over three years ago, I wrote a poem for him. My granddaughter has it framed and in his room. He was about six or seven weeks of age at the time. I was visiting their home and, of course, all my attention was on the baby. As I was talking to him and he was cooing softly, our eyes locked on each other, and he suddenly gave me a big toothless grin! My heart simply melted. It was his very first smile and he had given it to me!

The poem, written on January 24, 2015, is as follows:

Happiness comes to each of us in a different way. My great-grandson's birth enriched my life more than I can say.

This precious boy was born to one I love with all my heart. He's a first to all the family, and we adored him from the start.

His first name is Jon Ragan, and he's sweet as he can be. God created this perfect boy for all the world to see.

The baby and I were in his room on that cold winter day. I leaned down over him, speaking softly in my way.

He looked at me with knowing eyes as bright as they could be. That's when I saw the wondrous sight; Jon Ragan smiled at me!

He's seven weeks old, and I am eighty-three. At that moment time stood still when Jon Ragan smiled at me.

I've had many pleasures in my life, but none can ever be more touching and rewarding as when Jon Ragan smiled at me.

With tongue in cheek, I have some humorous advice for great-grandparents.

♦ No matter how adorable your baby is, try not to gloat to

your friends. They may have a great-grandchild whom they feel is the world's cutest baby!

◆ Share only a few photographs with clerks, nurses, doctors, and others. They do not have time to look at your entire album!

◆ The adventures and history you have lived through will be great to show later. Not while your grandchild is a toddler!

◆ Tight hugs and big kisses are more fun for you to give than for him or her to receive!

◆ Do not arrange to babysit for long periods of time. You will find that your energy level and endurance have "matured!"

It is true that great-grandchildren can learn a lot about life from us. However, we learn a lot about love from them. Enjoy him or her if you have a great-grandchild. If you look forward to great-grandchildren in the future, you will have an extra-special blessing when they come into your life and your heart.

CHAPTER FIVE

My Perfect Friend

This chapter is a tribute to Ginger Griffin, who passed away on March 2, 2002.

A plaque in my sunroom reads "A friend is a flower in the Garden of Life." I like it because it reminds me of how beautiful and fragile our friendships are.

Ginger and I had been friends for many years. Her husband was in high school with me in Valdosta. When they moved up the street from our home, we were all delighted. Now we could carpool with our kids, all of whom were around the same age. We did more than carpool. We became work friends as well.

When Ginger became the director of the Thomas County Service Center where I was a social worker, our friendship only deepened. We took trips to the beach together, shopped, and did lunch together. We gave each other's children's engagement parties when the occasion arose. Ginger even directed my daughter's church wedding, because I wanted her to do so. It was a first for her!

When we retired, the real fun began! We traveled and shopped in different towns around the Thomasville area. We were together at least three days a week. Whatever we did, whether it was antiquing, exploring, or just visiting, it always involved eating!

Our days together were so rewarding, laughing and talking, as we were very much alike. We were both Christians, loved God and family, our friends, our church, and each other.

The week before she died, we were in Tallahassee shopping for an event to be held at our church the following Saturday. When my phone rang early that Saturday morning, I thought it was Ginger telling me she was going to be late.

Instead, it was her son-in-law with the news that she had suffered a heart attack. She did not survive. People in Thomasville who knew her were heart-broken; she was loved by so many. Ginger was an outstanding role model for her husband, children, grandchildren, and friends.

The funeral service for Ginger was moving, beautiful, and uplifting. It reflected her life perfectly. The church sanctuary overflowed. Thankfully, my children came to be with me.

I think of Ginger every day, even sixteen years later. I remember her with joy and happiness. There are many memories of her in my house, pictures, cookbooks, cards, and more. She was a person that unselfishly gave of herself. She wanted others to have better than she had. She wore her faith like a badge of honor, touching many lives in her sixty-plus years. She especially touched mine. The friendship we had has enabled me to cherish and appreciate the special friends that I enjoy now. I try to give of myself to others just as Ginger did in her life. God truly blessed me with Ginger. I learned through her passing that time is fleeting. We must savor and enjoy now our special moments with those we love. Tomorrow is not promised to us. We need to be thankful to God when He gives us a blessing such as Ginger. I am a much better person because she was my perfect friend.

CHAPTER SIX

The Wonder of Faith

When I retired from my second career as a social worker at Legacy Village at Plantation Manor, a friend gave me a booklet entitled, *Bible Promises for You,* from the New International Version of the Bible (NIV). It has become one of my favorite resources when seeking guidance and reassurance.

In the foreword by Joni Eareckson Tada, she says, "The Bible reveals God's soul to us in a way that no other book is able to do. It is history, wisdom, and poetry."

God is the lover of our souls. He reveals His love to us when we study and believe in His Word. We all have problems, anxieties, worries, and frustrations. As I have grown older and more mature in my belief, I know without a doubt that my faith will sustain me through it all.

"The Lord is full of compassion and mercy," according to

James 5:11 (NIV Bible). This verse comforted me when life became difficult. He is with us always.

He tells us this in Jeremiah 29:12-14 (NIV Bible):

> *12 Then you will call on me and come and pray to me, and I will listen to you. 13 You will seek me and find me when you seek me with all your heart. 14 I will be found by you," declares the Lord...*

I was blessed to be raised by a Christian mother. I was in Sunday School and church each Sunday. My mother discussed her faith all the time. It was almost as though she had a special gift, but I did not fully understand it.

As the years went by, I was not able to grasp the meaning of her faith. I was still a Christian, believed in God, but the deep faith and complete and utter trust eluded me.

Years after my mother died in 1991, I faced the illness of my husband. Because dementia is such a slow and devastating disease, I, as a caregiver, become overwhelmed. I was lonely and frightened. It was at this point, my mother's faith in God became clear to me. Her faith helped her to cope with her problems. Now I needed her kind of deep faith to cope with mine!

On my knees, I asked God to come into my life and fill me with His presence. It was at that desperate point that I received this answer from His Word in Matthew 7:7-8 (NIV Bible):

> *7 "Ask and it will be given to you; seek and you will find; knock and the door will be opened to you. 8 For everyone who asks receives; the one who seeks finds; and to the one who knocks, the door will be opened."*

Words cannot describe the peace and comfort I received as I totally and completely put my trust and, yes, my faith in God. All my problems were still there, but now, I had my mother's kind of faith in my heart. I knew He would be with me and sustain me through anything.

So many times, we say or hear someone say, "I don't know how I would have gotten through it without the Lord." How true! My faith assures me that things are going to be all right no matter what happens. I am not alone, afraid, or unable to handle life's problems because of my deep faith.

I love God's promise in Joshua 1:9 (NIV Bible):

> *9 Have I not commanded you? Be strong and courageous. Do not be afraid; do not be discouraged, for the Lord your God will be with you wherever you go."*

CHAPTER SEVEN

Positive Thinking

RESILIENCE

Resilience is the ability to bounce back from a bad situation or event in your life. When we can recover from a minor setback, it prepares us for more traumatic events, such as losing a loved one, divorcing a spouse, or being fired from a job. I suggest practicing four habits to become more resilient.

1. **Be strong.** Do not give in to what is happening to you. We tend to over-react to bad news. Rather than thinking you will never recover or that your life is over, try to avoid extreme negative reactions that only make things worse. In life, most of the things we worry about never materialize. Always remember it is not what happens to you, it is how you react to what happens to you. Be strong in controlling your emotions and your behavior.

2. **Maintain proper perspective.** How is this problem going to change my life? How can I move forward and cause something good to result from it? The man in the story below was trying to be resilient!

> *An older couple were lying in bed one night. The husband was falling asleep, but the wife was in a romantic mood and wanted to talk.*
>
> *She said, "You used to hold my hand when we were courting."*
>
> *Wearily, he reached across, held her hand for a second, and tried to get back to sleep.*
>
> *A few moments later, she said, "Then you used to kiss me."*
>
> *Mildly irritated, he leaned across, gave her a peck on the cheek, and settled down to sleep.*
>
> *Thirty seconds later, she said, "Then you used to bite my neck."*
>
> *Angrily, he threw back the sheets and got out of bed.*
>
> *"Where are you going?" she asked.*
>
> *"To get my teeth!"[1]*

---

1   Author unknown. Senior Romance - Fropky.com, https://www.fropky.com/senior-romance-vt62263.html (accessed July 17, 2018).

3. **Take care of yourself.** When you are under stress, your body reacts negatively. Your immune system is not as efficient, your energy level drops, and your problem looms even larger. At this time it is essential to eat a healthy diet, get plenty of rest, exercise regularly, and avoid alcohol. The lady in the story below was trying desperately to get healthy.

> *"I feel my body has gotten totally out of shape. I got my doctor's permission to join a fitness club and start exercising. I decided to take an aerobics class for seniors. I bent, twisted, gyrated, jumped up and down, and perspired for an hour. However, by the time I got my leotards on, the class was over!"[2]*

4. **Ask for help.** It is not true that highly resilient people are stronger than other people. They are more likely to reach out to others when they need support and advice. Family and friends can be essential in the process of healing. When we have a sense of belonging, we can cope so much better. Seek professional help, if needed, through your church or family therapist. The man in the story below wanted to fit in with his friends.

> *Three men were sitting naked in the sauna. Suddenly, there was a beeping sound. The first man pressed his forearm, and the beeping stopped.*

---

2   Author unknown.

"That is my pager," he said, "I have a microchip under the skin of my arm."

A few minutes later, a phone rings. The second man lifted his palm to his ear.

When he finished the call, he explained, "That is my mobile phone. I have a microchip in my hand."

The third man, feeling decidedly low tech, and wanting to be a part of the group, stepped out of the sauna. In a minute he returned with a piece of toilet paper extending from his bottom. The others raised their eyebrows.

"I am getting a fax," he explained![3]

In summary, remember what happens to you is not as important as how you react to what happens to you. It is my sincere belief that we are all stronger than we think we are. What doesn't kill us will only make us stronger!

MEETING YOUR GOALS

A quote from Diana Scharf Hunt in *Reader's Digest's* book, *'Quotable' Quotes: Wit & Wisdom for Every Occasion,* states, "Goals are dreams with deadlines." Most of us have goals, dreams, and desires that we would like to accomplish during

---

3   Olson, Robin, "Three Men In A Sauna" - Robin's Web, http://www.robinsweb.com/humor/3men. html (accessed July 17, 2018).

our lifetime. A few of us write down our goals, then check them off when accomplished. Some goals are short-lived and simple, such as losing five pounds or making the perfect pound cake. Other goals are life-changing and complicated, such as accepting a new job or finding your marriage partner.

Setting a goal is the easy part. The real question is: Are you willing to accept the sacrifices necessary to meet your goal? Goal setting is also about the costs you are willing to pay. Many times when we fail even to try to meet our goals, we are frustrated, disappointed, and regretful. On the other hand, when we work hard and achieve a goal we have set for ourselves, we have a feeling of pride, accomplishment, and success.

An article on the website, "MindTools: Essential skills for an excellent career" (www.mindtools.com), lists five suggestions for meeting goals.

1. **Set goals that motivate you.** You must be passionate about it.

2. **Set smart, reliable goals.** Be sure the goal is attainable.

3. **Write down your goals.** Be specific. The act of physically writing down your goals is important.

4. **Have an action plan.** Include the necessary steps to meeting your goals.

5. **Stick to it!** Do not give up. Stay motivated

Goal setting is on my mind these days because I am working to meet a long-term goal of writing and publishing a book. Understanding the purpose of your long-term goal will help you to stay on track as you progress. My purpose in writing this book is to leave a legacy about life and living it to the fullest. I will be leaving a piece of myself for my children and their descendants.

My overall goal was to write a book entitled *It's Going To Be All Right.* My next step was to take my overall goal and break it down into smaller steps as objectives. I wrote down ideas and made notes, such as hiring an editor and researching publishers. My shorter-term goals became steps such as selecting the editor and writing one chapter at a time.

I made sure that I had a place to write without distractions. I needed a quiet environment to have total concentration. I wrote in the same comfortable, calming location each day.

If you are not in the habit of setting goals for your future, give it a try! You will be amazed at how helpful it is and how motivated you will feel to take that next step. Once you achieve your short-term or long-term goal, the fun part is rewarding yourself!

THE POWER OF LAUGHTER

We hear people say that laughter is the best medicine and there could be more truth to that than we think. In a *Psychology*

Today magazine article, titled, "The Science of Laughter," laughter is described as *the universal human vocabulary, produced and recognized by people of all cultures.* In the early field of laughter research, there is evidence suggesting there are health benefits that result in having a good chuckle.

Dr. Michael Miller, Professor of Medicine at the University of Maryland School of Medicine, is the author of *Heal Your Heart: the Positive Emotions Prescription.* Dr. Miller said, "Humor is so important that I place it as a daily requirement for a healthy heart, just like diet, exercise, and sleep. In fact, a good laugh will make you more likely to experience a good night's sleep, give you more motivation to exercise, and may even keep you away from unhealthy comfort foods that are often sought out during stress."

When you laugh, it sets off a chain of positive physical and mental reactions, according to Steve Wilson, psychologist, self-proclaimed "joyologist," and founder of World Laughter Tour. First, there is a dilation of your blood vessels. Your lungs take in more oxygen. Your muscles relax, which makes your digestion better. Your heart rate is elevated. Also, your brain produces neurotransmitters like endorphins.

Of course, a hearty belly laugh is not the only way to cope with negative emotions. Regular exercise, a balanced diet, and adequate sleep are all positive ways to deal with stress. However, laughter may be the most fun way to stay healthy. An excerpt from the poem, "Your Laughter," by Pablo Neruda, says it best: *Take bread from me, if you wish, take air away, but do not take from me your laughter.*

Need more reasons to laugh? Here are seven proven benefits for your body, mind, and social life:

♦ **You will feel less pain.** Pain tolerances become higher after laughter. Laughter releases endorphins which are natural pain reducers in the body.

♦ **You will experience less stress in your life.** Similar to exercise, laugher suppresses the release of stress hormones.

♦ **You will sharpen your brain.** Humor activates all parts of the brain at once. Laughter induces the type of brain waves that help with recall and memory.

♦ **You will feel closer to friends and family.** Most people love to be around a person with a good sense of humor. Being funny helps you make new friends.

♦ **You will lower your blood pressure.** A genuine laugh dilates your blood vessels, reducing blood pressure.

♦ **You will live longer.** According to a fifteen-year Norwegian study, published in 2016 in *Psychosomatic Medicine*, a sense of humor is positively associated with survival from mortality related to cardiovascular disease and infections in women, and with infection-related mortality in men. The findings indicate that a sense of humor is a health-protecting cognitive coping resource.

THE WONDER OF BEING A GRANDPARENT

Grandparenting is wonderful! I was never a "grandmother," I have always been "MeMo." When my oldest granddaughter was trying to say "MeMa," it came out as "MeMo," so that is what all five of my grandchildren and their friends call me!

Grandparents have time to do what parents do not have time to do. I have spent hours crouched behind a chair with my two-year-old Amanda having a pretend tea party! Children today have more modern expressions.

> A granddad asked his grandson to name our nation's capital. His reply was "Washington, D.C." When asked what the "D.C." stood for, the grandson said, "Dot Com!"

Children can, at times, try their grandparents' patience.

> An old man was grocery shopping with his grandson. The toddler was crying, and at times, screaming at the top of his lungs.
>
> As the old gentleman walked up and down the aisles, people could hear him speaking in a soft voice, "We are almost done, Albert...Try not to cry, Albert...Life will get better, Albert."
>
> As he approached the checkout stand, he carefully brushed the toddler's tears from his

eyes and said again, "Try not to cry, Albert...We will be home soon, Albert."

As he was paying the cashier, the toddler continued to cry. A young woman in the line behind him said, "Sir, I think it is wonderful how sweet you are to your little Albert."

The old gentleman blinked his eyes a couple of times before saying, "My grandson's name is John...I am Albert."[4]

Some of us will see our grandchildren grow into maturity and have children of their own. Great-grandchildren are a blessing!! Some of us have grandchildren nearby, others do much of our grandparenting by phone, mail, or texting, as I do with my three grandsons. Whatever the case, our tasks are all alike, to be a positive role model for our grandchildren, assisting them in being the very best that they can be.

Grandchildren keep us on our toes; we do not want them to think of us as old and boring. Years ago, my granddaughter, Amanda, asked me how old I was. I replied, "39 and holding." Five-year-old Amanda thought for a minute and then said, "How old would you be if you let go?"

A healthy sense of humor as we mature not only opens the hearts of our grandchildren, it enables us to live healthier and longer lives. One day, when my three-year-old granddaughter, Ansley, was sitting in my lap, she held my face in her hands,

---

4   Author unknown. Grandfathers? | Trap Shooters Forum, https://www.trapshooters.com/ threads/grandfathers.22071/ (accessed July 17, 2018)

looked intently at my upper lip and exclaimed, "MeMo, you are trying to grow a mustache!"

To love and be loved by a precious grandchild is the best and most rewarding feeling. Be the grandparent your grandchild needs you to be!!

Several of my ideas in developing a close relationship with grandchildren are listed below.

♦ **Give unconditional love.** "I may not like what you do, but I will always love you!" Unconditional love is the message our grandchildren must get from us.

♦ **Establish traditions**. Have a tradition that is special for each grandchild, just between the two of you. For example, I get a call from or give a call to my Ansley every night. She is always the last person I speak with before going to bed.

♦ **Establish trust.** Do what you say you are going to do. In our family, if you make a promise, you will keep that promise - no exceptions.

♦ **Take a sincere interest in their world.** Grandchildren will know when you are sincere about your interest in their lives. Meet and get to know their friends, if possible.

♦ **Compliment them when honestly deserved.** Show sincere approval.

- **Pass on your values.** Do so in a nonpreachy and nonjudgmental way. Grandchildren will learn from what you do, not what you say!

- **Listen, Listen, Listen!** Practice active listening.

- **Have a healthy sense of humor.** Share jokes and share secrets!

- **Model positive thinking.** Teach them to find something good about each day and to be thankful for the little things in life. The story of Attitude illustrates this idea perfectly.

> *Attitude was a woman who woke up one morning, looked in the mirror and noticed she had only three hairs on her head. "Well," she said, "I think I'll braid my hair today." So she did, and she had a wonderful day. The next day she woke up, looked in the mirror, and saw that she only had two hairs on her head. "Hmm," she said, "I think I'll part my hair down the middle today." So she did, and she had a grand day. The next day she woke up, looked in the mirror and noticed that she only had one hair on her head. "Well," she said, "today I'm going to wear my hair in a ponytail." So she did and had a fun, fun day. The next day she woke up, looked in the mirror, and noticed that there wasn't a single hair on her head. "Yea!" she exclaimed, "I don't have to fix my hair today!"[5]*

---

5   Author unknown. http://www.Spiritual-Short-Stories.com (accessed July 17, 2018).

CHAPTER EIGHT

Aging

HOW TO STAY YOUNG

For Christmas one year, my daughter, Beth, gave me a pillow with the inscription, "The heart is the happiest when it beats for others." These words are excellent advice if you want to stay young. Happy people do not have the best of everything. They *make* the best of everything!

Listed below are a few helpful suggestions on keeping youthful.

- ◆ **Cultivate happy friends.** Friends who are negative and unpleasant will bring you down with them. The man in this humorous story is not too cheerful.

  Gladys Dunn was new in town and decided to visit the church nearest her new apartment.

She appreciated the pretty auditorium and the singing by the congregation, but the sermon went on and on. Worse, it wasn't very interesting. Glancing around, she saw many in the congregation nodding off.

Finally, it was over. After the service, she turned to a still sleepy-looking gentleman next to her, extended her hand and said, "I'm Gladys Dunn."

He replied, "You and me both."[6]

◆ **Learn to enjoy the little things**. The more you appreciate life's simple pleasures, the more positive you will feel.

◆ **Surround yourself with the people or things that you love**. Whatever you enjoy most, whether it be your family, your pets, art, or music, spend time doing what you love. Enjoy often the people and things that keep you young.

◆ **Take care of your health**. Eat balanced meals and drink lots of water to stay hydrated. Get adequate sleep to feel rested.

◆ **Do not dwell on things over which you have no control**. Resiliency is the solution. There is a chapter in this book dealing solely with the ability to bounce back.

---

6   Author unknown. Dg Church Of Christ - Joke Of The Week - Gladys Dunn, http://www.dgchurch. org/jokes/g-h/gladys_dunn.htm (accessed July 17, 2018).

♦ **Seek to be of help to others.** Perhaps the advice on my pillow says it all. I believe that focusing on other people's needs keeps us young. When you reach out to others, you do not have time to focus on your own challenges. Helping others gives us a sense of purpose, accomplishment, and belonging. Now isn't that a beautiful thing?

HOW I GOT TO BE A HEALTHY 87-YEAR-OLD

When a person reaches the age of 87 and still has his or her physical and mental health, that is a true blessing! Although I feel great, I can relate to the following one-liners.

♦ *By the time a man is wise enough to watch his step, he's too old to go anywhere.*

♦ *Old age is when you have stopped growing at both ends and have begun to grow in the middle.*

♦ *Old age is having a choice of two temptations and choosing the one that will get you home earlier.*

♦ *A man has reached old age when he is cautioned to slow down by his doctor instead of by the police.*

♦ *Don't worry about avoiding temptation. As you grow older, it will avoid you.*

♦ *You're getting old when "getting lucky" means you find your car in the parking lot.*

♦ *You're getting old when you don't care where your spouse goes, just as long as you don't have to go along.*

♦ *Statistics show that at the age of seventy, there are five women to every man. Isn't that an ironic time for a guy to get those odds?*

♦ *Old age is when it takes longer to rest than to get tired.*[7]

Being a premature baby at three pounds, I guess I was born hungry and have tried hard to make up for it ever since! I do have a healthy appetite and eating is my favorite pastime. I have a friend who calls me "Chops" instead of "Betty!"

My mother was always health-conscious. She exercised with Jack LaLanne on television, took her vitamins regularly, and recognized the value of good mental health. I grew up knowing the importance of eating healthy, exercising, and having a good outlook. My mother would say, "Betty, when you worry, you get dark circles under your eyes!"

I did not want dark circles, so I learned at an early age to try not to fret and obsess over things I could not control. The following describes my typical eating pattern each day.

> *Breakfast*: I start the day with a bowl of cooked oatmeal mixed with oat bran and ground flaxseed. My son, Richard, calls this "Mama's slop." However, it does the job – energy for hours!

---

7   Author unknown. By The Time A Man Is Wise Enough To Watch His Step, He's .., http://www. haikuedhome.com/resources/OBSERVATIONS.pdf (accessed July 17, 2018).

Lunch: If I am eating out with friends, I relax my food rules. At home, I have a spinach salad with any meat or vegetables I may have on hand.

Afternoon snack: For over twenty years I have had a milkshake each day. The ingredients include:

1 cup plain yogurt	½ cup pineapple
1 frozen banana	1 cup frozen grapes
½ cup frozen strawberries	

Blend all ingredients in a blender until smooth.

Dinner: I am a big believer in having a well-balanced dinner. I prepare fish or chicken, fresh or frozen vegetables, and spinach or baked sweet potato at least three times a week.

Nightly snack: I like to eat something before bedtime (experts don't agree, but it helps me sleep). I call it my second supper, but it is just popcorn, yogurt, or even a sandwich. (I told you I eat a lot!) Believe it or not, I am not overweight.

Deep breathing exercises have been very beneficial to me. I began doing deep breathing techniques when my husband was ill. Deep breathing became a nightly routine, which allowed me to relax. I perform the deep breathing exercises the following way. Lying in bed on my back, I breathe in with my mouth closed to the count of four. I hold that deep breath to the count of eight. Then I breathe out through my mouth to the count of ten. I repeat these breaths ten times. Throughout the deep breathing exercise, I place my tongue on the roof of my mouth.

I must confess that I sporadically follow an exercise routine. I am, however, physically active - I move often and quickly. I do not sit still for long periods of time. I like aerobic exercise, which I learned to do lying on my bed to protect my joints.

In my opinion, good health is a balance of physical fitness and mental well-being. Living our lives is like dancing. We are not going anywhere, but we are enjoying the dance moves. Every day will not be perfect. However, there will be something in each day for which to be thankful. A positive attitude makes life worthwhile.

I do not smoke cigarettes or drink alcoholic beverages. I do not worry about my health problems. I turn them over to God and trust my physicians to take care of me. Working with people is a joy for me. Perhaps that is why I am an Ambassador at a lovely assisted living facility, Legacy Village at Plantation Manor. Life is good!

Everyone grows older, but everyone does not get old! As Norman Vincent Peale said in his famous book, *The Power of Positive Thinking*, "Live your life and forget your age."

The Sanity Test

A mental hospital was critically overcrowded. The doctor decided to get the patients seated in one large room to conduct a test to see how many patients they could discharge that day.

At the front of the room, the doctors took some chalk and drew a full-size door on a blackboard and offered an ice cream to any patient who could open the door.

There was a mad rush for the door, with the patients scratching and clawing at the door and handle.

The doctors were disappointed until they noticed a single patient who remained in his chair and was quietly chuckling to himself as he watched his fellow patients.

Encouraged that at least one patient could be discharged today, the doctors asked him why he wasn't trying to open the door.

The patient, who could no longer contain his laughter, shouted, "I've got the key!"[8]

AGE DOES HAVE ADVANTAGES

Many of you have heard Art Linkletter's famous quote, "Old age is not for sissies." I disagree with anyone who stereotypes those who are advancing in age. I like to think it is best to live your life and forget about your age because after all, age is just a number! Science keeps uncovering aspects of our health that do not get worse with time as much as we thought. Some improve with age!

---

8   Author unknown. Mental Hospital | Hot Jokes, http://hotjokes.net/mental-hospital (accessed July 17, 2018).

Age does have its advantages. One benefit of being in your fifties and beyond, is that you tend to make better decisions. "Older brains perform better in real-world tasks that involve decisions with long-term effects," says Darrell Worthy, Ph.D., Associate Professor at Texas A&M University. "That could be knowing when to ride out the wave in the stock market or organize a team at work."

Relationships become more meaningful to us as we grow older. People interact more with close friends than with acquaintances and find these close relationships more satisfying. Susan Charles, Ph.D., Professor of Psychology and Social Behavior and Nursing Science, at the University of Southern California, writes that older people rank their social and emotional wellbeing higher than younger ones. She states, "This is a big reason that you are better able to steer away from negative situations, particularly in relationships."

In researching for this book, I found interesting facts about people that prove we are never too old to learn new tricks.

> **Johanna Quaas** of Germany received an entry in the Guinness Book of Records as the oldest gymnast in the world in 2012. As of 2018, at the age of 92, she retains the record of the oldest gymnast in the world.

> **Jacquie Tajah Murdock**, a legendary Apollo Theater Dancer, at the age of 82, was one of the latest stars of Lanvin's Fall/Winter 2012 fashion advertising campaign.

Sister Madonna Bubar, an 87-year-old nicknamed "The Iron Nun," began completing the Ironman Triathlon when she was 52. She blasted through several age groups competing in Ironman races (a total of over 40). When she was 82 years old, she broke the age record again by finishing the Subaru Ironman Canada Triathlon.

Guess what? After 60 and beyond, allergies may affect you less. There is no scientific proof why the sniffles or watery eyes are less bothersome, but it means less seasonal misery for many. As we become older and more mature, we tend to appreciate the good things more. We may have different needs and remember places and events differently, but we can still enjoy life to its fullest. The group in the joke below believe in this philosophy.

A group of 40-year-old girlfriends discussed where they should meet for dinner. Finally, it was agreed upon that they should meet at the Ocean House restaurant because the waiters there had tight pants and nice buns.

Ten years later, at 50 years of age, the group once again discussed where they should meet for dinner. Finally, it was agreed that they should meet at the Ocean House restaurant because the food there was wonderful, and the wine selection was also good.

Ten years later, at 60 years of age, the group

once again discussed where they should meet for dinner. Finally, it was agreed that they should meet at the Ocean House restaurant because they could eat there in peace and quiet, and the restaurant had a beautiful view of the ocean.

Ten years later, at 70 years of age, the group once again discussed where they should meet for dinner. Finally, it was agreed that they should meet at the Ocean House restaurant because the restaurant was wheelchair accessible, and they even had an elevator.

Ten years later, at 80 years of age, the group once again discussed where they should meet for dinner. Finally, it was agreed that they should meet at the Ocean House restaurant because they had never been there before.[9]

NATURAL TECHNIQUES TO PREVENT AGING

Who does not want to prevent aging? Who would not choose to use natural techniques to achieve this goal? Exercise is of prime importance to staying fit and healthy, and it is one of the best anti-aging techniques. Physical activity tones muscles, helps to pump blood through the body and adds a healthy glow to the skin. Exercising for half an hour every day will help strengthen your mind and body.

---

9 Author unknown. "Here's To The Ladies Who Dine" | Huffpost, https://www.huffingtonpost.com/2012/03/22/heres-to-the-ladies-who-dine-joke_n_1373222.html (accessed July 17, 2018).

Another essential anti-aging technique is eating balanced meals. It is best to avoid strict diets and junk food. Meals should contain green vegetables and include fish in your diet several times a week.

Protect your skin to prevent aging. Harsh rays from the sun cause harm no matter the amount of sunblock that is applied. Avoid smoking and excessive drinking, as doing so causes the skin to look dull and flaky. Increase your water intake. Having seven to eight glasses a day will keep your skin hydrated and smooth. Water assists in the digestion process thus keeping the skin looking vibrant and youthful.

Meditation helps us to remain calm in the most stressful situations and positively affects our thinking and functioning power. You must complete your sleep cycle. Not sleeping affects the skin, causing it to lose its natural elasticity.

Who would not want to be mentally healthy as well as youthful looking? Resilience is the key. Chapter 7 includes the topic of resilience. However, it is worth mentioning here as well. Reducing stress in your life is an anti-aging technique. Less stress in your life leads to better sleep and reduces the appearance of age-related wrinkles and bags under the eyes.

Hopefully, these natural techniques to prevent aging will give you the strength to live life to the fullest, ready to face each new day with a sense of belonging and purpose.

A PATIENT'S EXPERIENCE
WITH KNEE REPLACEMENT

As a social worker at Plantation Manor, and later Legacy Village at Plantation Manor, I gave many tours of the facility. The tours involved much walking, which caused pain in my knees due to osteoarthritis. I had painful knees for many years. I tried postponing the worst of the discomfort by walking on the NordicTrack regularly, keeping my muscles and ligaments healthy.

There came a day in 2011 when nothing helped anymore. No amount of exercise, shots, or pain pills could ease the pain. At seventy-nine years old, I decided to have knee surgery as soon as possible! Surgery is required when one has "bad" knees. You reach a point when you know the time has come to "fix" them. After hearing so many horror stories about the procedure, I looked for a surgeon who would perform a double knee replacement to eliminate the need for a second operation. Double knee replacement surgery is no longer recommended, as the patient must be under anesthesia twice as long, which can cause complications.

In early 2011, my surgeon agreed to replace both knees at the same time. I am delighted to say for the past seven years I have had absolutely no problems with my "new" knees. They function as well as a natural knee would. Friends are both amused and annoyed when I perform my agility routine by putting my ankle on my ear!

Of course, no surgery is fun and knee replacement surgery

is a tedious and lengthy procedure. The part where your nurse, doctor, or physical therapist insists that you get up and walk on your brand new knees is particularly alarming, but you must obey! Straightening out your leg in the weeks to come is also a challenge, but eventually, you must do that as well. In my case, I was fortunate to go to an in-patient facility for ten days following surgery. I benefitted from intensive physical therapy for seven hours each day. My physical therapist was persistent and insistent. That combination made for real progress.

I was at home in two weeks and then had physical therapy on an outpatient basis. I was terminated from this after a couple of weeks because of the progress I had made. I must stress that the essential person in the recovery process is your physical therapist. They are there solely to help you achieve your goal. My therapists were all excellent, skilled, and knowledgeable.

The recovery period can be painful. In fact, exercising a brand new part of your body hurts! As I went through the process, I continually reminded myself how much pain I was in before the surgery. Every pain would be gain now because my knees were healing and would not hurt later.

Should you or someone in your life be facing this routine surgery, I have a few suggestions learned from personal experience.

♦ **Attitude**. A right attitude is by far the most important tip I can offer. When having knee replacement surgery, keep a positive, upbeat attitude with everything from preparing for the operation to graduation from physical therapy. Going into surgery knowing that you have decided to be pain-free is powerful. When the treatment gets intense, keeping your "eye on the prize" makes your physical therapy tolerable. I used a mental trick. I told myself going into the hospital that I was going to be the most successful patient they had ever had! Later I was told that the physical therapy department had never had a seventy-nine-year-old make as much progress as I had.

◆ **Physical health.** Be prepared healthwise before the operation. Eat well-balanced meals, exercise, and get enough sleep before going into the surgery. Healthy patients make faster progress after knee replacement.

◆ **Proper care.** At the appropriate time, the patient is told to use ice packs on the incision. I found that a small bag of frozen English peas worked much better than an ice pack. It conformed to my knee and could be used again after refreezing.

◆ **Reduced scarring.** When my knees were healing, I received permission from my doctor to apply shea butter to the incisions. The cream was moisturizing, reduced redness, and helped my scars to become smooth and barely visible.

◆ **Flexibility.** The knees must be kept flexible for an indefinite time after surgery. It has been over six years since my surgery. At eighty-seven years old, I enjoy an active lifestyle. I never sit for long periods of time without getting up, stretching, and moving around. I also practice aerobics in my home.

♦ **No pain, no gain.** Although this is a trite, overused expression, it is relevant when having one's knee replaced. The pain involved is worth the result of walking, standing, or sitting pain-free. I know this from experience!!

CHAPTER NINE

Dementia

TAKING A POSITIVE APPROACH TO ALZHEIMER'S DISEASE

No amount of positive thinking can prepare one for the journey of caring for a loved one who has Alzheimer's disease. Walt, my husband of forty-five years, began showing signs of dementia approximately eight years before his death. The disease progressed at a rapid rate until he died in 2002. News of having someone you love diagnosed with this terrible illness is devastating and overwhelming. My goal in life is to help those whose loved ones are going through the stages of dementia. I want family members to know that they can survive the trials that lie ahead. Making a difference in the lives of family members is extremely helpful to them and rewarding for me.

My first recommendation is to urge the caregiver to seek all available resources for the Alzheimer's disease patient as early as possible. Resources may be in the form of consultation with health experts and diagnostic testing to determine courses of treatment, such as medication and specialized daycare.

My doctor recommended a book to me when Walt first became ill, *The 36 Hour Day,* by Nancy L. Mace, M.A., and Peter V. Rabins, M.D., MPH. The book tells almost everything one needs to know about dealing with dementia. I failed to follow his recommendation until much later. Had I read *The 36 Hour Day* when I first learned of it, I would have been more knowledgeable and better prepared for the stages of the disease.

According to the National Institute on Aging, legal, financial and medical experts encourage people recently diagnosed with a severe illness – particularly one that is expected to cause declining mental and physical health – to examine and update their financial and health care arrangements as soon as possible. To ensure that the person's late-stage or end-of-life decisions are carried out, the following documents are available:

1. <u>Advance directives for health care</u>, such as a living will, durable power of attorney for health care and Do Not Resuscitate order.

2. <u>Advance directives for financial and estate management</u>, such as a will, durable power of attorney for finances, a living trust, and decisions about organ donation.

3. <u>Guardianship and conservatorship</u>, if necessary, for those deemed unable to make their own decisions.

The caregiver must make it a priority to care for themselves physically, spiritually, and mentally. Remember, you are not useful to anyone if you are ill or burned out. I was fortunate to have supportive friends and a loving family. I learned to lean on them. The primary caregiver can expect feelings of depression and of being overwhelmed. Joining a support group can be a helpful way to share feelings. Take one day at a time and be resilient. I found relief watching funny shows on television. I desperately needed the humor that I found in them, and, surprisingly, my husband enjoyed them as well.

Empathy is essential. You must try to see things as the dementia patient sees them. I found out that my husband responded to affection. Hugging, touching, holding hands, and saying "I love you" were helpful. We would attempt to find humor in frustrating situations. For example, there were numerous times then Walt would put his clothes on backward, put my clothes on, or refuse to put his shoes on. Of course, not every act is funny. In some situations, I found that redirecting, interrupting, and distracting him worked.

A person with dementia is usually unable to respond emotionally to the caregiver by expressing appreciation or affection. Nothing can be done to make the patient realize how much the caregiver is giving and how little the caregiver is receiving in return. The caregiver must realize this as merely another characteristic of dementia.

The dementia patient has a short attention span, which is an advantage to the caregiver. It is best to follow routines and keep them simple. Do not argue with the patient or expect them to be reasonable. I learned that it is natural and healthy to become angry at times. I also learned that there is no place for guilt in any situation. If and when you do become angry and lose your temper, it is to your advantage to forgive yourself and move on. Do the best you can do; that is all you can do. One positive aspect related to loss of memory is the patient does not remember later that you lost your temper and spoke harshly!

My husband suffered from frequent hallucinations. The hallucinations frightened and upset us both. During these episodes, I learned to comfort him by saying that I did not see what he was seeing. However, I assured him that I knew that what he was seeing was real to him. I assured him that everything was going to be all right. Then I would redirect his attention to something else.

BEHAVIORS OF ALZHEIMER'S DISEASE

Dementia is the severe loss of mental ability. Many diseases, all of which affect the brain, cause multiple aspects of memory loss and abnormal behaviors. Some of the most common diseases that cause dementia are:

1. **Alzheimer's disease** Most common diagnosis; loss of nerve cells in the brain due, in part, to amyloid plaques

2. **Vascular dementia** Second most common diagnosis; due to strokes that damage blood vessels in the brain

3. **Dementia with Lewy Bodies** Due to abnormal deposits of protein in the cortex of the brain

4. **Frontotemporal dementia** Due to abnormal formations, nerve cell loss, and degeneration of tissues in the frontal and temporal parts of the brain

5. **Parkinson's disease** A movement disorder, where muscles are affected and dementia may develop

Other causes of dementia include organic brain syndrome, depression, drug use, and thyroid dysfunction. A person may have more than one disease in which each causes dementia, such as Alzheimer's disease and vascular dementia.

In the six or so years my husband, Walt, had dementia, he exhibited many disturbing behaviors. I am going to discuss these behaviors in this chapter. Of course, this disease involves communication. The following joke is about miscommunication.

A man and his wife were driving their RV across Florida and were nearing a town spelled Kissimmee. They noted the strange spelling and tried to figure out how to pronounce it — KISSa-me, kiss-A-me, kiss-a-ME. They grew more perplexed as they drove into the town. Since they were hungry, they pulled into a place to get something to eat.

> *At the counter, the man said to the waitress, "My wife and I can't figure out how to pronounce this place. Will you tell me where we are and say it very slowly so that I can understand?"*
>
> *The waitress looked at him and said, "Buuurrrgerrr Kiiinnnning."[10]*

In caring for my husband, I learned three things that helped both of us.

1. **Distract.** When Walt became agitated or disturbed, I distracted him by drawing his attention to things like helping with a task, eating a snack, or watching a television program. When I quickly changed the subject, he forgot about being upset.

2. **Deflect.** At times, Walt, due to his disease, would be intent on doing something that was destructive or that could be harmful to him. Those were the times where deflection worked. I gave him an interesting alternative to what he was about to do. I did it any way I could!

3. **Stay calm.** If I became upset, Walt would become more upset. Entering their world by expressing positive emotions to them calms them and keeps you calm as well!

One of the most annoying and challenging behaviors my husband exhibited was extreme paranoia. He accused me of

---

10   Author unknown. "Joke of the Week," | https://rvtravel.com/rv-travel-newsletter-issue-804/ (accessed July 17, 2018).

everything from stealing to infidelity to lying to throwing away his possessions. I had to realize that he lived in a world where each moment was starting over. He had no memory of what went on beforehand. When he would say, "You have stolen my dentures."

I would not say, "You lost them."

I would say, "I'll help you find them."

I found by distracting Walt and remaining calm, we could better cope with each episode of paranoid behavior. There were many each day.

Another behavior characteristic of dementia is agitation and aggression. Again, distract as best you can. Use a calm tone always. Medication can help with this type of behavior.

Clinging behavior is a characteristic of someone with dementia. My husband followed me around and, at times, would not let me out of his sight. The caregiver must remember that the patient is in a strange, frightening world, where he or she feels alone and helpless. When possible, I enlisted the help of others to come in and give me a break. Also, I tried to find activities he could do alone to keep him occupied.

With Walt, there were many complaints with which to deal. For example, my husband would accuse me of hitting him, being mean to him, or being a stranger to him. I would, again, distract and deflect, while remaining calm. I found these techniques worked best for me.

Walt would frequently hide things. The best way to handle this behavior is to remove valuables and dangerous items from your home or lock them securely out of view.

It is important for family members to remember that the dementia patient does not do any of these things to intentionally hurt them. These behaviors are symptoms of the person's illness. My time as a social worker was valuable to me as a caregiver for Walt. I knew it was not my husband saying and doing hurtful and upsetting things. I was always aware of the behaviors being symptoms of his illness.

Walt had the classic "sundowning" behavior, which means his symptoms became more pronounced in the late afternoon and evening. He wandered at night which is typical behavior of persons with dementia. I tried to keep Walt active during the day so that he would be tired at night. I also made sure that he went to the bathroom before bed.

Other unpleasant behaviors would come and go. One was repeating the same questions over and over. Ignoring this behavior and avoiding answering Walt's questions would make him angry. I learned to use whatever response worked for me at the time.

In addition to repetitive questions, Walt repeated actions. I controlled this by giving him something to do that made use of this behavior, such as selling peas, counting change, or folding towels.

Shouting or using profanity was out of character for

Walt because he had never done this before his illness. Unfortunately, this is a common behavior of persons with dementia. Their inhibitions are gone. His profanity was an embarrassing problem with which to deal.

Hallucinations were frequent in the course of my husband's illness. They began early on before any other symptoms appeared. One day, out of the blue, Walt said, "Do you ever think Beth and Richard are here with us?"

I explained that our children lived out of town, so I did not think they were with us. I remember thinking his question was odd because we had not yet considered a diagnosis of dementia. As the disease progressed, the hallucinations became more vivid and more frequent.

He "spoke" with our son, even though he was not present in our home. He fought imaginary dogs in our yard and fought fires that were not burning. Through all of this, I learned to say, "Walt, I know you believe what you are seeing, but I do not see it. Just know that it's going to be all right."

Please remember the person with dementia is not doing any of these things to hurt you. In fact, it is he or she that is hurting the most. Love, patience, and faith got me through the nightmare of dementia. I am blessed to be an optimist and I instinctively feel that "this too shall pass."

The joke below clearly defines the difference between an optimist and a pessimist.

Two friends, one an Optimist and the other a Pessimist, could never quite agree on any topic of discussion. One day the Optimist decided he had found a good way to pull his friend out of his continual pessimistic thinking.

The Optimist owned a hunting dog that could walk on water. His plan? Take the Pessimist and the dog out duck hunting in a boat.

They got out into the middle of the lake, and the Optimist brought down a duck. The dog immediately walked out across the water, retrieved the duck, and walked back to the boat.

The Optimist looked at his Pessimistic friend and said, "What do you think of that?"

The Pessimist replied, "That dog can't swim, can he?"[11]

POSITIVE WAYS FOR CAREGIVERS TO COPE

I coped in positive ways by looking for and finding something good to come out of a challenging situation. I learned not to give up when I still had something to give. I learned not to be afraid to encounter risks. It is by taking chances that we learn how to be brave. I did not let myself dismiss my dreams. To be without

---

11   Author unknown. "The Optimist and the Pessimist," | http://www.backwoodshome.com/irrev-erent-jokes-issue-86/ (accessed July 17, 2018).

dreams is to be without hope and to be without hope is to be without purpose.

I found good things coming from my experiences. I learned to appreciate the little things. I found and focused on something positive that happened each day. For example, a smile or laugh from Walt, an unexpected pleasure or event, or a glimpse of a happy moment from the past. I held onto anything that made me feel better, even if only for a brief moment. In looking for the good in a difficult situation, I found parts of myself that I did not know existed. I grew in ways that I never expected.

I will never forget what happened the day that we moved Walt to an assisted living facility. It was with much apprehension, fear, and trembling that I drove him to Plantation Manor. However, I was happy and relieved with what happened next. We walked into his room in the dementia wing and I explained, "Look, Walt, your room looks just like a hotel room." He suddenly grabbed me, smiled and exclaimed, "Well, let's get it on!"

During this time, I found my faith in God strengthened. I have been a Christian for many years, but through this experience, I found out just how much God works in our lives. Prayer kept me going. I prayed for strength and received the strength that I needed. God does not promise that we will live a problem-free life, but that through having problems we will learn to lean on Him. I now know how true that is, because He was with me through each trial that I faced. The Bible, my church, and my Sunday School class gave me something to lean on. To help me get through each day, I relied on God first, then family and friends.

Remember God will not put more on us than we can bear and "this too shall pass." Philippians 4:13 (New King James Version Bible, NKJV) became my motto: "I can do all things through Christ who strengthens me."

I found the way I handled stressful situations impacted others. My family, particularly my children and grandchildren, took their cue from me during this time. Because my behavior influenced them, I tried to set a good example by maintaining a positive outlook. Family and friends said they were better able to face small problems, after seeing how I handled more significant problems.

My ability to deal well with my stressful situation had the bonus of my feeling good about myself! My self-esteem increased and healthy self-esteem means more help for others. My husband was a kind and gentle man who was loved and revered by his family and respected by his friends. It means so much to his memory that because of him, I am committed to helping people be the best they can be.

MORE CAREGIVER ADVICE

Many caregivers feel that people do not know what they are going through unless they have gone through it themselves. They are so right! The caregiver for a dementia patient is truly a hero. Volumes have been written and countless words spoken advising on caring for the caregiver. These resources are all well and good, but I know from experience that nothing makes the pain go away!

The caregiver is tired, frustrated, and under extreme stress. In my work with caregivers, I have found that many will repeatedly struggle with a feeling of guilt. Guilt is an emotion that never helps the situation and brings the caregiver down to a new low. Although guilt is common, it is a wasted emotion.

Prayer worked for me when I felt guilt over my situation with my husband. There were times I lost my temper with him. That was the time I asked God to forgive my actions, give me the patience to stay calm, and control my emotions. One blessing with caregiving for a dementia patient is they do not remember that you were angry with them. It is only human to lose one's temper at times, especially when dealing every day with the distressing behaviors of someone with dementia. If temper outbreaks occur frequently, it is best to seek the help of a trusted professional.

Speaking of help, all caregivers need a break from caregiving. Research has proven that taking care of yourself as a caregiver may save your life. It is estimated, according to a Stamford University research study, forty percent of caregivers for Alzheimer's disease patients die before the person in their care. There is a term used by the medical community: caregiver syndrome or caregiver stress syndrome. The chronic stress of caring for someone with dementia can cause depression, anxiety, and anger, as well as health problems, such as high blood pressure and a weak immune system.

Support groups are helpful for families going through this experience. I recommend a support group for all family members with a loved one with dementia. Something as simple as planning an activity once a week that you enjoy will allow time for yourself. Whether it is taking a long walk, having lunch with friends or attending a social event, it will help you greatly.

Below is a portion of the letter my younger granddaughter, Ansley, wrote. I presented the letter at the Dr. Jim Neill Memory Walk for Alzheimer's Awareness, held on April 11, 2015.

"The fact that you are all here today implies that you each in some way have been affected by this horrible disease, and for that, I am truly sorry. Today, I want to address the grandchildren of those who have Alzheimer's disease. I have only one piece of advice. Do not shy away from your loved one with Alzheimer's disease.

"It is not the confused glances or the heartbreaking realities that I remember when I think about Papa. It is the rare moments of clarity; the books he read to me when I was little; the stories I heard one hundred times and still asked to hear again; Memo and I picking on him at night when he would fall asleep in the chair watching television; Papa making the same bet with me every time I saw him, just so he would have an excuse to give me a dollar; randomly honking the horn and saying 'there was an ant in the road;' eating breakfast with him at Hardee's on Saturday morning; and always letting me get away with murder, because let's face it, I was his favorite.

"If I were to think back, I could recall any number of instances related to his Alzheimer's disease that were not pleasant, but those are not the memories that pop into my head on a daily basis and make me smile. My sister and I are blessed to have had this remarkable man for a grandfather. I hope you will follow my advice and spend as much time as possible with your grandparents, no matter how heartbreaking. A small amount of sadness is well worth a lifetime of joyful memories."

My final advice to a caregiver of someone with dementia is the experiences you encounter, both good and not so good, can be helpful to someone else in the same situation. The sharing of this information is an opportunity for help and healing for all involved. What better to offer someone in need than to give your experience, your support, and your love?

CHAPTER TEN

Words of Cheer

My third great-grandmother, Elizabeth Esabella (Eby) Touchstone, was a remarkable woman. She was still writing in her journal at age 108. A quote from her journal, dated November 13, 1885, is as follows: "My husband, Solomon, lived to be 90 years of age. I have always said that time does not measure life as much as life measures time."

Collecting words of encouragement and inspiration have lifted me up and sustained me throughout the years. Enjoy the following quotes and pass on the good cheer!

"We make a living by what we get, but we make a life by what we give."

- *Sir Winston Churchill*

"Success is the ability to go from one failure to another with no loss of enthusiasm."

- *Sir Winston Churchill*

"If you can spend a perfectly useless afternoon in a perfectly useless manner, you have learned how to live."

-   *Lin Yutang*

"Always be kind, for everyone is fighting a hard battle."

-   *Plato*

"Happiness depends upon ourselves."

-   *Aristotle*

"The foolish man seeks happiness in the distance. The wise man grows it under his feet."

-   *James Oppenheim*

"You can make more friends in two months by becoming interested in other people than you can in two years by trying to get other people interested in you."

-   *Dale Carnegie*

"Don't judge each day by the harvest you reap, but by the seeds that you plant."

-   *Robert Lewis Stevenson*

"Always laugh when you can, it is cheap medicine."

-   *Lord Byron*

"The robbed that smiles steals something from the thief."

-   *William Shakespeare*

"Of all the things that wisdom provides, to help one live in happiness, the greatest by far is the possession of friendship. Eating or drinking without a friend is the life of a lion or a wolf."

- *Epicurus*

"Twenty years from now you will be more disappointed by the things that you didn't do than by the things that you did do. So, throw off the bowlines, sail away from the safe harbor, and catch the trade winds in your sails. Explore, dream and discover!"

- *Mark Twain*

"You cannot do a kindness too soon, for you never know when it will be too late."

- *Ralph Waldo Emerson*

"Keep your fears to yourself, but show your courage."

- *Robert Lewis Stevenson*

"Ideas are like rabbits - you get a couple and learn how to handle them, and pretty soon you have a dozen."

- *John Steinbeck*

"Age does not protect you from love, but love, to some extent, protects you from age."

- *Jeanne Moreau*

"Don't judge each day by the harvest you reap, but by the seeds that you plant."

- *Robert Lewis Stevenson*

CHAPTER ELEVEN

Positive People = Positive Influence

Throughout all our lives we have people who make an impact on us, people who mold and shape us, who affect our future behavior and our character. My father, Cecil Emory Spell, was such a person. In my formative years, his honesty, hard work, and faith in God had a positive effect on my life. He loved people and had a desire to help others. I wanted to please him and to be just like him.

My maternal aunt, Kate Louise Whitaker, was also a positive influence throughout my life. She adored me and I adored her. She was giving of herself, loving, and always made me feel special. I believe God used her to brighten my world, which increased my self-esteem and sense of security. Later in life, I had a very dear friend, Ginger Griffin, in whom I saw Christianity in action. Her positive outlook and her faith influenced my life. Another friend whom I love dearly is Gail Lancaster. She and I worked closely together at Plantation Manor, which is now Legacy Village at Plantation Manor. I believe that without Gail's inspiration and confidence in me, the support group would not have been as successful. Gail has been a positive, loving, giving, encourager!

God has truly blessed me with a loving Christian family. My two children, Beth and Richard, lead successful lives and I could not be more proud of them. Beth is an amazing daughter, who is always there for me. She was my rock during her Dad's illness. I have said many times to many people that I would never have coped as well without Beth by my side. She does much more than love and protect me, she is an experienced and accomplished Chief Executive Officer of two mental health centers and has a busy and rewarding life in Americus, Georgia. We are very close and talk every day. I am thankful for this closeness and secure in her love for me.

Richard retired from the Georgia State Department of Transportation. However, he is hardly retired as he is busier now than ever at his own company. He is an extraordinary son. Richard is brilliant, talented, and artistic. I admire him and love him very much! He is just a phone call away and is always there when I need him.

Beth is married to Allen Ragan, my dependable and wonderful son-in-law. They have two children, Amanda Ragan Ritter and Ansley Ragan Evans. They are my loves! These two girls fill my heart with love and my life with joy. They will also tell you that they love their MeMo (that's me!).

Richard and his lovely wife, Kristan, have a son, Aaron. He is handsome, sweet and charming. Kristan has two sons,

Walker and Cooper Powell, giving me a total of three terrific, fine-looking grandsons!

I could not have asked for two more incredible grandsons-in-law than Tony Ritter and Chip Evans. I am their MeMo too! As I am writing this book, my great-grandson, Jon Ragan Ritter, is three-years-old. He is the son of Tony and Amanda. He is the light of all our lives!

It is interesting that each time I speak to any of my family members, "I love you" is their closing remark. These dear people inspire and motivate me to be the best that I can be. I deeply feel the importance of setting a good example for them. It is how we live, not what we say, that inspires people. From the time Ansley and Amanda were babies, we prayed together. These are still some of my most precious memories.

CHAPTER TWELVE

Final Reflections

M y purpose in writing this book is to share my thoughts in hopes of inspiring, uplifting or just reminding readers to stay positive. We all have problems - we face hardships, we lose loved ones – no one is exempt. It is often stated that it is the hardships of life that form our true character. A couple of phrases from Tracy Lambrecht's book, *Nothing Stays Buried*, are meaningful to me:

> *"Grief is the cost of love."*

> *"Even if your heart is broken, the love inside the shattered pieces never dies. It can lift you up, or it can drag you down."*

As I have lived these 87 years, I would like to share with you a few things that are important to me.

♦ **Strength.** "I can do all things through Christ which strengthens me." Philippians 4:13 (King James Version

Bible, KJV) This Bible verse is my motto, and I have proven it over and over again throughout in my life.

♦ **Generosity.** Give expecting nothing in return.

♦ **Kindness.** BE KIND!! I try to show kindness wherever I am. When I am in public, if a person looks sad, upset or bored, I find a way to give him or her attention. The compliments are sincere and range from complimenting their smile to admiring their jewelry. It is a blessing that this small effort on my part can bring confidence and pleasure to another person. Kindness is free and is so rewarding for the giver and the receiver. I hope that you appreciate and enjoy the little things. I love the words of wisdom by Mamie McCullough, author of the book, *Get It Together and Remember Where You Put It*:

"As we treat others, so in time they will become."

♦ **Caring for others.** Focus on and be interested in other people more than in yourself. Be happy for other's good fortune.

♦ **Happiness.** Life is to be enjoyed. Be yourself; be happy.

♦ **Prayer.** God can handle all your problems. Pray about every worry and concern. Give it to God and trust him to handle it.

♦ **Resilience.** How I respond to a situation is more important than what happens to me.

♦ **Authenticity.** Be authentic. Not "put on."

♦ **Mindfulness.** I know now that where my mind goes, the body follows.

♦ **Appreciation.** At my stage in life, I feel if I worry, fret, and am in a bad mood, I am wasting a day. I focus on something good every day.

♦ **Love.** Let others know you love them. Don't wait until it is too late to tell them.

♦ **Discretion.** Don't share your most personal family problems with friends. You will forget the problem, but they will always remember.

♦ **Self-care.** Reward yourself frequently! I am very good at rewarding myself after my accomplishments, such as chores completed or a productive day.

♦ **Gratitude**. Be grateful always. Life is so full of beautiful, amazing things and incredible people to love. Never take anything for granted.

♦ **Problem-solving.** I have learned and am affirming every day that there are many ways to look at a problem or a difficulty in my life. I can view it as a challenge, an opportunity, and a learning experience. Many times it turns out to be a blessing in disguise. When I was much younger, I worried needlessly and now I turn problems over to God.

◆ **Legacy.** Don't save material things for a rainy day; tomorrow is guaranteed to no one. Today is a gift; that is why we call it the present. As we age, we become aware of who will remember us and for what reasons we will be remembered. Your love, loyalty, and faith are what will live after you are gone, not the material things.

◆ **Self-giving.** "Love is when the other person's happiness is more important than your own." H. Jackson Brown Jr.

◆ **Protection.** "Have I not commanded you? Be strong and courageous; do not be discouraged, for the Lord your God will be with you wherever you go." Joshua 1:9 (New International Version Bible, NIV). This is one of my favorite Bible verses.

◆ **Support.** I have known for a long, long time that friends and family are essential to my being happy and fulfilled. I am blessed to have had both a loving and caring family and friends who are like family. They all bring me joy and fill my heart with love.

My family members and the people mentioned earlier in this chapter are the most positive influences. However, they are not the only ones who have a positive effect on my life. My close friends, whom I love dearly, are so important to me and such a blessing. We talk on the phone, go out to lunch or dinner, and we have been known to go on many "adventures" (when we go on out-of-town day trips)! When something good happens to one of us, we celebrate. When the news is not good, we feel our friend's pain and pray for them.

I have been a member of the same women's Sunday School class for over fifty years. There is a sense of continuity and belonging, as well as a strong bond of love and fellowship with the members of the class. Through the years, some of our members have passed away. We miss them, pray for their families, and always remember them fondly.

I have a plaque a friend gave me years ago. It states, "A friend is a flower in the garden of life." So true!

As you or I go about our daily life, we can influence or be influenced by people with whom we come into contact. There are some wonderful, inspirational people in this world. Be on the lookout for them and give or receive a blessing!

If you have made it this far in my book, Congratulations! You are at the end!! I pray you found something interesting and helpful inside. Thank you and may God bless you!

Afterword

I turned 60 years old on my last birthday. Southern women, particularly those from my mother's generation, have an unspoken understanding that age is never voluntarily revealed, and if one must disclose "how old" she is, the number is to be lowered considerably. Not my mother. She readily discusses her age as a badge of honor representing a life filled with many accomplishments. Having a close, personal relationship with God, laughing often, preparing and eating wonderful meals, spending lots of time with family, enjoying a wide variety of close friends, and finding joy and peace regardless of circumstances are her measures of a life well spent. Her dedication to strive for success in the things that really matter and her desire to use her experiences to inspire others to do the same motivated her to write this book. "It's going to be all right" are words that I've heard my entire life. I've used them often and hopefully will continue to grow in my belief of them. Yes, I'm 60. Not quite yet a badge of honor but I'm confident that with faith, time and a great role model I'll get there.

Beth Sawyer Ragan

About the Author

Betty Sawyer is a Georgia native and has lived in Thomasville for over fifty years. She holds a Bachelor of Science Degree in Social Work from Valdosta State University. She retired from the State of Georgia in 1995 after thirty years of service. After her retirement from the State of Georgia, Betty served as Director of Social Services at Plantation Manor Assisted Living and Memory Care Community for fifteen years. Currently, she serves as Ambassador for Legacy Village at Plantation Manor.

She is the mother of two, grandmother of five and great-grandmother of one. Betty cared for her husband at home for over six years as he suffered from dementia. He passed away in 2002.

As a result of this experience, she founded the Alzheimer's/Dementia Support Group at Plantation Manor in 2003. The group was to become the largest and most well-attended gathering of its kind in the State of Georgia (according to the Alzheimer's Association of Georgia). For her efforts with the group, she received the 2007 Horizon Award, presented by the Alzheimer's Association, Georgia Chapter, for her advocacy in the fight against Alzheimer's disease.

The Dr. Jim Neill Alzheimer's Walk is a local Thomasville event named for Dr. Jim Neill, an area physician who diagnosed himself with the disease. Betty served as an organizer for the successful fundraising event for twelve years. She was recognized by the Red Hills Gerontology Association of Thomas University for Excellence in Education and Advocacy in Caregiving.

An accomplished author and speaker, Betty is a popular keynote presenter for organizations, agencies, colleges, and universities interested in dementia and topics related to gerontology. Because of her service to her husband, her extensive experience in social work, and her professional training, she is uniquely qualified to inspire and give hope to others.

CPSIA information can be obtained
at www.ICGtesting.com
Printed in the USA
LVHW032201271018
594840LV00001B/4/P